My Life With Psoriasis

The story of what finally worked for me and kept me clear for over 30 years

By: ROSS GAMBRIL

Dedication

This book is dedicated to all of you who have suffered the slings and arrows, the trials and tribulations and the incredible mental anguish that this devastating affliction has caused you.

It is my wish and hope for you that that this book and the information in it can possibly change your life in the way that it has changed mine.

Table of Contents

Introduction

This book is a labor of love. One that is dedicated, from the bottom of my heart, to each and every one of you who have had to endure the pain, the incredible suffering and embarrassment that this disease inflicts on us. It is not a long book, like most that are out. It just has the basic information in it about what I did to conquer psoriasis and hopefully enough information that will help you make an educated decision on whether or not to try what worked for me.

After I had stayed virtually 99% clear for over 3 years, about 31 years ago now, was when I first wrote about my struggle to clear my psoriasis. Since that time, I have experimented and researched as much about psoriasis as I possibly could and this book includes all of the additional information that I was able to gather since that time.

To my knowledge, there is no one who I am aware of, who has been able to stabilize their psoriasis in virtually total remission for the length of time that I have been able to, for over 30 years. There may be some others. I have been told by some, who have read my first booklet and used what I described in it, that they were able to achieve the same results. There may be others who may have stumbled across what I have found. I have no way of knowing that. It is only after being able to stabilize the condition for that period of time was I able to have any substantial, valid and meaningful observations to pass on. Those observations, that are based on my personal experience, are what is in this book. Take them for what you think they may be worth. What I found out literally changed my life.

We are among a group that is two percent of the world's population who have it. There are even more, three times as many, who suffer from eczema. The reason that I believe it has never been in the forefront of medical concern, in my opinion, is for two reasons: 1) it's not life threatening, although it does dramatically change your life; and 2) it's not mentioned to outsiders much, by those of us who have it, because of the embarrassment that we endure.

After three years of using this treatment and having it work so wonderfully, I came to the point that only I noticed that I had it. I then realized that I could not, in all clear conscience keep it to myself so, I did write a short booklet that described my journey to become virtually totally clear. This book is a rewrite of that original booklet and it has everything that I have learned about psoriasis since I became clear. The simplicity of what I did and still do to this day and the way it works so wonderfully is both a fantastic joy and a serious irritation. Why, you ask, is this treatment that I found so irritating? Because psoriasis has been around for well over 2,000 years, most likely since the beginning of time, and no one has discovered this treatment, until now! It has literally changed my life.

Most of the books that I have read and I've read a few, have obviously been written by people who don't have it, at least the ones that I've read. It seems that whenever you read any of the books that are written by those supposed experts, they sound more like a classroom lecture rather than someone just trying to tell a real story to anyone who has it and knows how serious an affliction it is. None of us deserve that from anyone, much less from someone who hasn't experienced it first-hand. I sincerely hope that this book and my writing in it reaches you in the right way and doesn't sound demeaning or belittling in any way. It is not intended to be. It's just my story and the story about what I found that worked and still works incredibly well for me today.

This book is about my experiences as a psoriasis sufferer but, what I found out is also very relevant for those who suffer from eczema, since both psoriasis and eczema are somewhat related. Much of both are very similar. Virtually everything that I've written in this book is very relevant to both those with psoriasis and eczema, with the exception of the scale and the arthritic problems that occur with psoriasis.

The information in here is everything I've learned over 50 years. As was once titled in a movie, I've learned "The Good, The Bad and The Ugly". It's all very, very real and is my own personal experience with this incredibly devastating condition, psoriasis. It is what I have found using myself as the guinea pig. What's in this book will only make any real sense to those who suffer from it too, either psoriasis or eczema. Those who don't may just find it as an interesting read and nothing much more.

I sincerely hope that this information is as valuable to you as it has been for me.

About the Book

The following body of work has been written as non-fiction. The events which have been described by the author are expressed to the best of his knowledge and recollection. All in all, it is a peek into the author's life in dealing with psoriasis and the associated occurrences, so there is bound to be subjectivity. It is the truth, as comprehended by the author, and not some fiction that is made up for writing this book. The book has been written with the awareness of the disease and humor of the author's overall experiences, as well as a few particular experiences.

1

My Psoriasis Journey

It was 1996, when I first decided to write a booklet about my experiences, having become clear of any outward indications of having psoriasis for about 3 years. At that time people would tell me to sell my book or, that I should put it on the Internet for free. The problem was that most people believe, and they are right to some extent, that free advice is worth what you pay for it. With this book, I have rewritten the original booklet to include all the additional information that I have found in the 30 years since becoming virtually clear. I'm doing it my way and I hope to not only share my past experiences with you but, to promote what I have come across and also explain to you about its effectiveness. I also hope to promote what has come to be Psorclear™ as a viable, effective and consistent treatment for not only psoriasis but, also an effective treatment for eczema and other related skin conditions.

I have written this book from my experiences as a psoriasis sufferer for over 50 years and my perspective of what I have experienced. It is a first-person account, my account, not an abstract observation of the condition, as is the case with most books that are out. I also make references in the book to eczema, which is a very similar condition although it does not manifest itself as severely as does psoriasis. The primary difference between psoriasis and eczema is that eczema does not develop into scaling skin, nor does it affect bone joints. The redness, the itching, the general discomfort, the visual embarrassment, as well as the psychological trauma that they both cause which are, for the most part, virtually identical for most.

I won't get rich from publishing this book but it will cover my costs and I will get this information out to those of you who need it and deserve it. Many individuals, even those who have only recently contracted it, are unfamiliar with the condition of psoriasis. Some believe it may be infectious. It is NOT. A person's skin cells merely develop at a much faster rate, incredibly quicker than normal skin cells. This results in a build-up of scaling skin on the skin's surface that, as you well know, causes serious irritation and inflammation and which can be incredibly debilitating in extreme cases, especially with psoriatic arthritis.

It is not and I repeat, is NOT curable, at least not at this point in time. Hopefully someday it will be. For now, all any of us can do is treat the outward indications of it in the best way possible. What I have found is the way that has worked the very best for me of anything I've ever tried and hopefully it will work for you too. Although the medical community is well aware of the information that is in this book, it is most likely that this information will never come out on their end, since it is not economically feasible for the medical community to do so, which I will talk about later in the book. Most psoriasis patients like you, describe their experience as managing the outward symptoms, adapting to the limitations created by the disease and dealing with the incredible psychological trauma that we all have to deal with. We don't tell others about it and we use incredible effort to just try to get by the best we can. We hide that we have it from everyone we can.

The information in this book is much more valuable than its cost but, my sole intention is to share with you the information that was given to me, along with what I found out as time progressed. It also includes what I've learned from my experiences and my findings, as well as how and why I decided to finally have what is now Psorclear™ formulated.

There are many psoriasis sufferers who probably won't purchase this book because they think, given how much their treatments have cost them, that anybody who is giving this knowledge for free, on the basis of any cost comparison, cannot possibly have anything valuable to offer. Unfortunately, those people are wrong. There are those who will think that this is just another treatment concocted by someone who has never had it themself. They too are wrong and misguided.

There are those of you who, although you may only have a very minor case of it and are somewhat dismissive of the fact that it's there, should read this book to find out what I have found to be true about psoriasis. It just may be of some help to you too, if only to help you to understand how bad it can be and for you to be thankful that it's not that bad for you.

I suffered from this condition, just like you do, for over twenty years before I discovered this treatment. The memories I have from that time of how horrendous it was will never disappear, and those related experiences are unforgettable, no matter how much I try to forget. Those vivid memories are what gave me the motivation to write this book. I also realize that I will always have it, even though it has virtually disappeared now and it has been like that for a very, very long time. I will never be able to forget my past.

I'm not going to keep you in suspense for much longer. I'm sure there are those of you who are interested in learning what it is I use that was and continues to be so effective for me. This product is currently marketed under the trade name Psorclear™ and has totally changed my life for the good. It is nothing more than a common mineral supplement that is found in daily life that has been specially formulated to substantially minimize or, in the majority of instances, as well as it did in my case, virtually completely eradicate any outward signs of having it. It has also been formulated to substantially reduce or eliminate any of the known unpleasant potential side effects from using it.

Throughout the following Chapters, I will provide you additional information on how Psorclear came to be and how it was developed. Some of you may not have the patience to read the whole book, so skip forward to Chapters Three and Four. However, please take the time to read the complete book. How Psorclear™ itself came into existence is described completely in Chapter 5 of the book.

I have explained in full what I did, with the help of a friend who is a genetic researcher, in order to accomplish the outcome that I have achieved. To find out what those results have been and continue to be to this day, you must read this book in its entirety. I've also discussed the results of my considerable research, experimentation and studies that I have conducted over the last 30 some years.

If I was to tell you that salt enhances the flavor of potatoes, you may not believe me until I show you how much salt to use or, in this instance, how much of what I used for my psoriasis and what worked best for me. What's more significant, in this instance, is that you may not achieve the same results as I did without the knowledge I have gathered and am passing on to you in this book.

This book is an account of what my good friend, the genetic researcher, suggested and what I did as a result of her advice. It is based on the information that she provided, as well as what I discovered in my research findings. This information is not meant as a medical recommendation in any way, shape or form, as I am not a physician and thus cannot legally provide any kind of medical advice, nor would it be reasonable for me to do so. This is all about my own life experiences as they relate to my having psoriasis, which I believe that I have a responsibility to share with you in order to possibly help to improve your life.

In my professional life, I am a real estate developer who happened to have a friend who works as a genetic researcher at a major medical center, who was aware of my condition and was concerned about it. She shared her thoughts with me about my psoriasis and I then took her suggestion and ran with it.

The choice is yours whether or not you want to follow my lead. It is entirely up to you whether you want to consider its significance as valuable to you. Nothing more than what I did and what I discovered in my research can I relay to you. I can only convey what I was told to me during those times. In this book, I will share with you all of the additional knowledge that I have obtained, as well as some of the many experiences that I have had over the last three decades.

To keep things simple, while still providing you with information about my experiences, I have attempted to relay what I have been told and what I have discovered from my thorough study of this dreaded disease. I could write much more and go into more depth, but I'll refrain from doing so for the purpose of being as concise as possible. To be honest, there are far too many books out there that are hundreds of pages long and were written by individuals who have never experienced what it’s like to suffer from either psoriasis or eczema and have no idea what it's like to actually have it. I did not include any of my psychological experiences in this book. I don't think I have to remind you of what you're going through right now.

As we all know, it’s absolutely devastating and way beyond the imagination of those who don’t have it. As for how I'm feeling right now? Normal, and I mean that in a good way! All the outward signs of having psoriasis are now gone. If you have any further questions after reading this book, please do not hesitate to contact me and I will do my best to answer them as quickly and as best as possible.

The word Psoriasis is a derivative of the Greek word "psora" which means "to itch". Psoriasis, to my knowledge, is the oldest disease on the face of the earth for which there has never been any meaningful, effective treatment that works consistently... until now. About forty years ago, I was told by a Catholic priest that there are biblical references to lepers and their white scaled lesions. That makes the disease, by my guess, well over 2,000 years old.

There have been records of individuals suffering with psoriasis since the beginning of recorded history and three books of the Old Testament in the Bible include passages regarding people who suffer from psoriasis. One book, Leviticus, is entirely devoted to people who possessed scaly skin that was red and white in color. Additionally, it is referenced in the Books of Numbers and Kings. They were referred to as lepers in those days. Guess what? Lepers do not have scaly skin that is red and white but, those who suffer from psoriasis do. Leprosy is not white. Instead, it appears as dark colored lumps on the skin that may severely distort a person's body parts. As you may or may not know, when psoriasis appears, it first appears as red spots, then with white scale and people who had psoriasis during that time, were most likely exiled to Leper colonies. That was, without question, a terrible sentence for those individuals. I would assume that the worst that any of us have ever experienced pales in comparison to what those unfortunate individuals had to go through.

Psoriasis does not have any gender, race, or age distinction, nor does it have an ethnic distinction but, some research has indicated that in certain cases, it seems to be more common in women than in males. Other studies, on the other hand, have shown that it is more common in males than in women. You will learn about psoriasis and the different theories that are in this book, as well as discover the many contradictory ideas, theories and research that exists about it. This is what makes it so tough for us and doesn't help our situation. Nobody in the medical community seems to have a definitive answer for the condition of either psoriasis or eczema.

Psoriasis, the disease that you and I suffer from, is not unique by any stretch of the imagination. Psoriasis affects about two percent of the world's population, with over an estimated 7 million individuals in the United States alone suffering from it. There are a lot more people who suffer with eczema, more than 3 times as many, which is extremely similar to psoriasis in both its appearance and symptoms, which I stated earlier. Severe cases of eczema tend to show as blisters, not scaled skin. There are numerous opinions about what the origin of the condition is and the circumstances that may cause your skin to flare up, but there are a few factors that are generally agreed upon. A person's immune system is associated with it and that it has a genetic origin. The chance of having psoriasis may skip as many as two generations or more.

As stated earlier, psoriasis is essentially a condition in which skin cells multiply at an astronomically higher rate than normal skin cells, resulting in red patches, the white scaling of dead skin and the inflammation, not to mention overall discomfort. Normal skin cells regenerate about every 23-28 days. It is comparable to, but considerably more severe than, eczema in terms of appearance. There are no diagnostic tests for psoriasis, no blood tests that can be performed. Diagnosis is done visually, and many individuals may be suffering from it without even realizing it until they are informed by someone else or by a dermatologist. I was completely unaware of it until it was pointed out to me by someone who was well-versed in the subject.

As I stated earlier, there isn't any cure, I repeat, NO CURE for either psoriasis or eczema. I will undoubtedly repeat this several more times in this book because, it is very important that you fully understand that. There seem to be many, many people who have it and who seem to think that there is a cure out there somewhere. As of now, there is Not one. Instead, there are just treatments to reduce the visible external symptoms of the disease. It is not infectious in any way. Psoriasis may go into remission on its own and remain in remission for a long period of time.

Usually, remission lasts between one to twelve months, but in some instances, it may last for longer periods of time.

There are eight basic types of Psoriasis;

(1) Plaque Psoriasis, the most common type.

(2) Guttate Psoriasis.

(3) Pustular Psoriasis.

(4) Erythrodermic Psoriasis.

(5) Inverse Psoriasis.

(6) Scalp Psoriasis.

(7) Nail Psoriasis.

(8) Psoriatic Arthritis.

It is possible to have only one or all eight types at the same time, and they can affect the various areas of the body at the same time. At one point, I was completely covered and had it virtually all over my body. Thank God, I've never had to deal with psoriatic arthritis. Speaking with others who have or, are currently experiencing that, I've learned that it is extremely painful and, in many cases, becomes physically immobilizing. It goes without saying that, as a male, I don't have any concept of how debilitating and psychologically traumatizing this disease can be for women and girls. I can only understand and sympathize with what you're going through. It is beyond my understanding regarding how mentally devastating it can be for you. I'm not sure I can fully comprehend it myself. To the females reading my book, please accept my heartfelt sympathy and I hope that this book may be helpful to you and change your life the way it did mine.

I understand that you suffer with either psoriasis or eczema, and that many things I say in this book may not be necessary for some of you to hear. It is possible that some of you have had similar experiences to mine, and that some of you have had even worse experiences however, it is also possible that some of you have only recently (within the last two or three years) come down with this affliction and are not yet aware of the extent of what it can develop into.

I've tried to write this for everyone and to be as honest as a person who has psoriasis can be about their experiences. The majority of you may not need, or even want to hear my story. Although, many of you may just be like me when I first developed it, reliant on what you are told by others, both in and outside the medical community. We all have been given so many different types of treatment recommendations from those who have not personally dealt with it other than to treat its symptoms.

There is a definite distinction between those who have experienced it first hand and those who are, for the most part, outsiders and onlookers. Unfortunately, most in the medical community fall into the latter category. Many of you may already well know, it affects various areas of the body in different ways, and I have personally experienced them all, again with the exception of psoriatic arthritis. In any event, I have done my best to provide you with my discoveries and their effectiveness, as well as specifics about what I have done to maintain my current condition.

Up until the point where I found what worked, I was informed of the various treatments that were commonly used to treat my psoriasis. All of the information that I received, possibly information that you have been given too, is based on medical studies that have been performed on groups and the caveat that "we're not quite sure" is always attached. Until now, there was no common denominator that made any sense to me in all the information I had received.

Please do not take any off-the-wall humor that may occur in this book personally. I will do my very best to keep it to a minimum. In no way is it an effort to make light of psoriasis or the pain that it causes. It's not humorous in any way, shape or, form. I simply find it amusing how some of the most horrific events that have occurred to me now appear almost comical in hindsight, since they have passed and I am no longer in the same situation.

With all my heart, I hope that you will get the same advantage from this book as I received from both the knowledge that was given to me many years ago and the information that I have found through my research, in the years since then. Then hopefully you may, as I do today, look back on your experience and find some humor in the physical and mental agony that you are going through right now. I now consider myself to be in all practicality, free of psoriasis, despite the fact that I know I will always have it. I am overjoyed that, after all these years of suffering from this excruciating disease that I have finally discovered something that not only works for me but, that I can also share with you as well. I am grateful to my friend for pointing me in the direction of this discovery. I always suspected that someone would eventually figure out what was really effective. It has worked and continues to work wonderfully for me, and I really hope that if you decide to give it a try, it will work for you as well.

It is my hope that this book will help you understand my condition at the time, what I did due to my friend's suggestion and how it has virtually eliminated my psoriasis. I hope you will find this book helpful. You may even be able to connect my experiences to some of your own personal circumstances as a result of this.

2

The Hard Times

I've been a sufferer of psoriasis for over fifty years now, fifty-four to be precise. It was the final week, first semester in college when I came down with it. I didn't even know what it was until a fraternity brother of mine told me. His mother had it. At the time, it started as small patches on my elbows and I really didn't think anything of it. Little did I know what was just beginning to happen.

Over the next couple years, I became almost covered with it, over 85% of my body. It spread to my arms, legs, my entire torso (front and back), hands, feet, finger nails, hair, inside my ears, on my face and yes, even on my genitals (talk about effectively killing a sex life that had not even started). When I scratched at it and it itched horrendously, as you well know, it would most likely start bleeding. It did provide a draft deferment for me to avoid going to Vietnam, which I can honestly say I was not happy about. You see, I was in line for pilot training through college R.O.T.C., until I flunked the physical because of it and my dream of being a commercial airline pilot was dashed to bits. For someone who had all these wonderful plans about my future and what I wanted to do, this situation left me utterly devastated. I was ashamed of my skin and my condition and it kept growing worse. I thought that maybe that was it for me, and my good days and great dreams were gone.

At one time, and that "one time" lasted several years, I had scale so bad on the front and back of my knees and elbows that when I bent my arms or legs, the skin would crack and start to bleed, not to mention the unbearable heat that was generated from the lesions. Skin inflammation, cracked skin and bleeding had become my “new normal”. Every evening, before I went to bed, I would coat my body and my scalp with whatever medication was working the best at the time, be it a cream, a lotion or, an ointment. I would completely wrap myself in cellophane, from head to foot every evening, complete with a shower cap (lovely night wear, huh?) and then go to bed. Wrapping with ointments was not recommended by my dermatologist but, sometimes it was the only way it would work. My situation would get so much worse that if I didn't put on these ointments, I really didn't have a choice in the matter. When I went to bed, I was more hermetically sealed than a fifty-dollar cigar. At one point, I even thought that someone should develop and market a washable, zippered cellophane night suit for psoriasis sufferers.

Each morning, I would spend the first half hour or so, scraping the scale off of my body with a very sharp knife, just to make it through another day. This was my daily routine. Then I'd do it again the next night. I would then take my trusty dust buster and vacuum the scale off of my bed that came from the unwrapped parts of my body. It seemed more like I was sleeping on a beach than on a bed. It sure helped to lessen my desire to want to spend any time at the beach, which helped since I couldn't wear a swimming suit. I hated the obnoxious stares and repetitive questions I would get about my situation.

For over twenty years, I never wore shorts, short sleeve shirts, nor did I ever go swimming. Not being able to go swimming really hurt the worst, since I used to swim competitively, before this situation. My cousin was the 1984 U.S. Olympic Swimming Team coach. I loved to swim and did so whenever I got the chance. I even had a job at a local swimming pool at one point, but after I came down with psoriasis, I could not simply take off my clothes. People would look at me and sometimes get very uncomfortable.

On one occasion that I remember very well, I had gone to a car wash where they washed the outside and cleaned the inside of the car. When I got out of the car, the attendant asked me if I had just come back from the beach. I said yes. I didn't want to get into a discussion about that stuff on the floor of the car being scale that I had scratched off of my legs. It's not really their fault, they just don't know and I could understand. Even with all I have gone through, I am thankful each and every day, that I am not one of the two percent of us who suffer with psoriatic arthritis. I honestly can't even imagine what that is like and my heart goes out to those of you who do.

My reason for telling you all of this is not to try to impress you in any way, or gain your sympathy. God knows, I could find a better way. I know that I'm not telling you anything that you don't already know. After all, you bought this book because you are going through something similar to what I was and are looking for a better way, something that might really help, just as I was. I want to relate all this to you, just so that you realize that, yes...I have dealt with this, that I understand your pain and I empathize with your situation.

I'm also relating this to you so that you realize that the information in this book comes from the first-hand experience of having the affliction, my using of the available prescriptions and other treatments. More importantly, the change in my condition that occurred when

I started my treatment to control it, which will be fully described in the later chapters. This is a true story. The story of my life and the condition that I have spent decades of my life dealing with. I was my own guinea pig and am giving you a first-hand account of that experience.

Everyone I have ever met who knew that I had "something", had a home cooked or, half baked "cure". This applies to not just those of us who suffer from psoriasis or eczema but to many who may suffer from other skin conditions that one can have. People like us have always heard an old wives' tale or, what their friends or, what relatives have suggested or, what they had read on the internet.

People like these don't really understand the situation and what you're going through, even though it might be coming from good thoughts and feelings and with good intent. They sure didn't have a clue when it came to what I was going through at the time. It got to the point where I had heard the same "home remedy" ideas so many times that, whenever someone asked the inevitable question about what I had, my somewhat warped mind would take over. I would answer their questions with slightly twisted statements describing my condition that I'd rather not repeat here. The repetitive nature of these questions became mundane to me and so my sarcasm would often take over.

My very warped responses usually did stop any further conversation about it though. Someone once said to me, "Those who know, know...those who don't, don't matter". The context here is that if you have it, it matters to you, if you don't, you don't have a clue. It's just a reason for those other people to ask silly questions about it and make "useful" treatment suggestions.

Face it, unless you have psoriasis or are in the medical field, chances are you can't even spell it. Can't blame them, not the easiest word to spell. Some can't even pronounce it properly and I remember it being once referred to as "sorry asses". Those people have no idea how really right they are. We are exactly that, unfortunately.

What people don't realize is that hearing about things like that don't make us feel better, not in any way, shape or form. Just like all the happy, peppy psoriasis commercials that are now on TV. That's because they don't know, nor do they really understand, what it's like to have it. They may not have the capacity to understand the personal pressure it creates just by having it, the incredible itching, the pain, the massive scaling, even bleeding in a lot of cases, the deformation of fingernails, toenails, the scaling scalp, the suffering and the incredible embarrassment, as well as the serious psychological issues that come along with it. Not to mention getting all those questions from those who aren't the least bit aware of what it is.

They don't realize the effort that we all have to go through just to hide it from others, just to avoid getting those well-meant but misguided questions. Not everyone is like that, some people are more empathetic than others and really do have the capacity to understand the pain of another. Having said that, it is a rare breed that actually has that capacity. It's actually human nature that most of us will just ask and then shed light on almost anything without considering any and all of the issues involved. We all tend to have our opinions, no matter in this case, how misguided they may be.

Then along comes my friend, with information that I thought finally did have some credence and validity to it and something that really made sense, for the first time since I got this stuff! Even the dermatologists I've been to and I've been to some who are said to be world renowned in the field of dermatology, both in Chicago and at the Mayo Clinic, who only just merely treated the outward symptoms with medications that were nothing more than a temporary solution.

When I went to the Mayo Clinic, I actually knew more about psoriasis than the dermatologist who I talked with did. It was actually a very surprising and upsetting experience. I guess you never learn a lot about it as merely an onlooker. They really didn't have a clue as to what the cause was. At least if they did and I suspect they just might, they didn't bother telling me. Why not? Your guess is as good as mine but, economics might be to blame.

They just treat the symptoms, even to this day. After all, all it does is cause discomfort, extreme discomfort but, it isn't life threatening. There are about 9,600 practicing dermatologists in the US at this time. Of that group, like with us, probably only 2% of them have psoriasis and really know what it's like to have it. Do the math. That's about 190 of them. The chances of you finding a dermatologist who really has first-hand experience is slim to none. The rest only know about what they've studied, read or observed, primarily using us as their guinea pigs for experimentation purposes.

As for the homeopaths, they have their ideas about natural treatments and diets. Unfortunately, they too are just as misguided as the medical doctors, knowing what they've observed and read but, not actually having experienced it. Such as in life, often people talk about topics they have no experience in, and we listen. The analogy that I can use here is me trying to tell a woman what it's like to have a baby and to tell her about the misery she'll go through while carrying the child.

I'm a man. How would I know what it's like to give birth to a child? I will never experience what it's like to give child-birth. I can only relate what I've been told and what I've read. I have seen some childbirth movies as part of being a dad and going to childbirth classes with the mother of my kids but, in reality, what do I know? So, now to make the long story short, I know virtually nothing, having never experienced it first-hand. Just like 98% of the practicing dermatologists who advise us about our condition, who give us their thoughts, opinions and who use us as their experimental guinea pigs. For the most part, as we have all unfortunately come to find out, what they offer us is only from second hand experience and, in reality, almost totally worthless. What they offer works for a while and then they try something else on us.

My first trip to a dermatologist was in 1967. He was a very nice man and I have to give him credit because he was totally honest with me and said that they didn't really know much about the condition. He did tell me that I wouldn't be drafted into the military but, I already knew that. He said it is hereditary and could skip generations, which was the most baffling thing for me to comprehend.

No one in my family (on either side) had it and I wondered, "why me?" Why did it have to be me? As it turned out, my father ended up having a bit of psoriasis crop up in his scalp at the age of 54. Over the next twenty years, my treatment costs including office visits, averaged well over $100.00 per week. That was over $100,000.00 back then, if you're trying to get an estimate. That’s over $600,000 in today’s dollars (2021), based on the value of money back in 1970. Insurance only covered a portion and later on none at all, due to it being a "pre-existing condition".

I was a very willing guinea pig at Northwestern Medical Center for the development of what was to become Diprolene, as well as a couple other “new” medications. The everyday expenses were piling up on me and so I did that to help keep the treatment costs down. Trial products come with the obvious catch of nothing being certain, and so you are on the edge at all times. Anything could happen.

The other part of that experimental process is that you must literally sign your life away, absolving those doing the testing of any responsibility if something should, God forbid, go wrong.

I've used coal tar treatments, which didn't work and just made me and my hair smell bad. I have been on all the topical steroids, at one time or another and have suffered from TSW, Topical Steroid Withdrawal. I used to keep two to three different types in my medicine cabinet because, sooner or later, the one that I was currently using didn't work anymore and I would have to switch...again. I've been on the psoralens for use with UVA and UVB (they made me sick). I have used methotrexate and that was a scary experience. Having to be monitored like something could go wrong at any minute was a scary thought.

At the time I didn't know what it was. The minute that I found out what methotrexate really was, I took myself off of it. What methotrexate does and why it's used for cancer chemotherapy and to treat psoriasis is that it will drastically inhibit the reproduction of rapidly reproducing cells. However, it is non-discriminatory and will attack all rapidly reproducing cells in your body, like blood and hair cells, as well as a host of others.

I'm sure some of you have known someone who's gone through cancer chemotherapy and lost their hair while they were on it. I've had steroid injections, used Tegasin and "the latest toy on the shelf" at that time, Dovonex. I tried anything and everything, whatever could help me become normal again and hopefully become the man that I used to be. I would have some hope each time I tried something new, but sadly, the hopes always faded when the lasting results weren't there.

We have all tried one treatment after the other, after the other and before you know it, you've tried nearly everything with little to no hope and options for a better future, in effect, disappear. Most of you are like how I was, just hoping and hoping that something would finally work. A lot of you who end up in this situation just accept your fate and try to go on with life, using products to help control your situation the best that you can. I kept on trying, kept doing my best to find whatever solution that might be offered and tried my best to manage my condition, but nothing worked. Nothing worked until I found what I found.

What all the other treatments have in common are:

1) They are all regimented protocols that take concerted effort to maintain.

2) Most have side effects that can cause serious health problems, especially the oral and injected medications.

3) The minute you stop using the medication or, with prolonged usage of the same medication (not even that prolonged), it will, most likely, flare up again worse than when you first started using it.

That is what happened to me when I used the topical steroids. Probably like you, it made me wonder what was actually going on.

With the "new" biological products like Stelara, Cosentyx, Otezla and the others, as with the other stuff, it will decide when it wants to stop working and eventually it will stop. Like with other prescription medications, your body will, most likely, eventually build up a resistance to them. I'm sure there of a lot of you who have already experienced that and know more about those medications than I do. I'll get into more about the biologics later in this book.

How many times have you used something that you thought worked great, only to find out that it suddenly stopped working, a week, a month, even a year later? And, when it stopped working, the psoriasis seemed to come back even worse than before, the flare-up's kept getting worse. According to what I was told at the time, there is an explanation but, no one has ever explained it in a manner that ever made real sense to me. In the following chapter I'll tell you what I did find out all on my own.

I've been through it all and have used everything that has ever come out in the market, except for the biologics and the "new" generics, which are just the same medications that I had already used years ago, before the patent rights expired. You see, all generic medication is, is a prior medication that was developed and patented by a particular company whose patent rights have expired and is now being produced by other companies.

The other companies are free to copy the formulas and produce the medications at a much-reduced cost, due to the fact that they have absolutely no research, development nor approval costs to deal with. That works for simpler products like aspirin and cold remedies but not for medications for such a complex condition like psoriasis or, eczema. If it didn't really work for us years ago, it won't work for us today. Supposedly all the research and technology has created improved products, except for one thing, they are still only to treat the symptoms, not the cause.

It's very much like putting a new coat of paint on a wood boat. If the boat has dry rot, it makes the hull look nice for a while, but it does nothing to fix what's causing the paint to keep blistering and flaking off. And, the minute you stop painting the boat, the dry rot and paint flaking comes back, even worse than before...sounds like psoriasis to me.

What you must come to grips with is the fact that there is No Cure for neither psoriasis nor eczema and there, most likely, will never be one. I am sorry to have to break it to you this way, but I am sure you somewhat knew this to be true. You will always have this condition and you need to realize full well that that is the case, no matter how badly you wish it wasn't.

All any of us can do is treat it to keep it under control and hopefully substantially reduce or eliminate the outward indications of it existing. All those who profess to have found a cure are, for lack of a better word, phonies. They are, in effect, snake oil salesmen trying to get you sucked in as another customer (oops, sorry, I mean patient) with another treatment that only masks its visual effects. Those treatments will only work for a while, as you by now well know. The product that I had formulated, Psorclear, treats the cause of the affliction and, while doing so, also drastically minimizes and, in some cases, totally eliminates any outward signs of it even existing. You could finally become what you so badly want to be...just a person with normal skin!

As I said earlier, neither psoriasis nor eczema are life threatening diseases. Since it is not economically feasible to for anyone to find a cure for either one, neither doctors nor the pharmaceutical community will most likely come up with the ultimate cure we all hope to find. I hope I'm wrong but, I don't think I am. I've had decades of experience with this affliction and I'm pretty sure that I know what I am talking about.

Here's an analogy. In the early 1800s, until the mid-1950s, polio was very devastating and, in many cases, there was up to a 30% chance of a fatal outcome. It is a disease that affects the central nervous system and could cause both internal (organ) and external (muscle) paralysis. Both doctors and drug companies made millions, maybe even possibly billions of dollars treating patients who had this and were suffering from this condition.

One day Dr. Jonas Salk came along with a vaccine that has since almost totally eradicated polio from the face of this earth. To my knowledge, there has only been one case known to exist in the US since the late 1970s. This was a good thing because polio was such a devastating affliction that affected millions of people all over the world, just like psoriasis and eczema. The major difference here is that polio could be fatal but, neither psoriasis nor eczema is. All those who treated patients with it and who supplied treatment medication for it suddenly, after about 20 years, were out of a job.

That won't happen with psoriasis and eczema. They will do their best to keep the patient base, you and me, appeased with treatments that will work for a while and will only treat the outward symptoms, not the cause. The last thing any of them want is to lose any of their regular, good paying customers (oops, I mean patients). Dermatologists don't really make money from removing lumps and bumps. Once they're gone, so are the patients. That doesn't happen with us.

We're actually nothing more than the guinea pigs they need to keep trying new stuff on. They have absolutely no motivation to find a cure for us. The real money is in just treating the symptoms. We're the ones who end up suffering from the lack of motivation for them to really find something that will really help. It actually does make a bit of sense when you think about it but, it sure doesn't really help any of us. You have to continue going to them to find some solution, or, to at least maintain a better condition. And then, there are those of us who seem to gravitate to internet support groups to hopefully find help. I'll write more about than later. You have no other place to go, and so you are stuck in this spiral. But, not anymore!

3

The Good Stuff

OK, let's get to what it is that I use and why I've been told that it works.

Like I said earlier, I was told that I should start taking zinc. The readily available zinc supplement tablets that can easily be found in any pharmacy, health food store, most supermarkets, even in some department and discount stores. However, they have their drawbacks and shortcomings. That's why Psorclear was formulated, specifically to eliminate what I had found to be those drawbacks and shortcomings from taking common zinc tablets. In the next chapter, I will tell you exactly how I started taking it, the amount of what is now Psorclear I that I took and, to this day, am still now currently taking. I will describe how my skin became, for the most part, clear as well as the results I saw as I had become clear. Also, I will tell you about the formulation of Psorclear and why it was formulated in the way it is. Yes, even what the one side effect is that I have found and what I do to combat it. It is not a serious one at all. Finally, what I have discovered to be the biggest individual causes of flare ups, although it just confirms what a lot of us have always suspected.

I do still have them, only now they are almost totally insignificant and I am the only one who really notices. To everyone else it just looks like a little, bitty skin rash or imperfection, that is even if they notice it at all. I have found specific causes for the flare ups that I had, which has helped to minimize them tremendously. I never really knew specific causes of flare ups, probably like you, because of the way the other medications worked and then didn't. You try and try to figure it out but, no matter what you do because of all the different medications you try, something always seems to cause a flare up and sooner than later you start wondering if you'll ever be able to determine the cause. Some people do figure out what causes the reaction, but as you well know, it’s different for everyone. I have never been on any other treatment that has remained so effective for this long in my life, other than Psorclear. It's been about Thirty years now. Long enough that I was actually able to discover the causes and effects, related to my flare ups. What I've actually been able to do is substantiate some of the theories that exist and question even more some of the others. I’ve also been able to make complete sense out of some of the stuff that I heard and read, and probably, like you, have found a lot of the stuff to be totally nonsensical.

Psorclear is the only treatment that I use and it is not a cure. Maybe someday there will be one. All we can do is hope. What I found out is that, what is now Psorclear, is the most effective, the easiest, the least expensive and by far the safest treatment for psoriasis that I have ever used.

For the rest of this chapter, I'll relate to you what was told to me regarding the reason to take zinc, which is what I took in tablet form in the beginning. It will probably make as much sense to you, as it did to me. There are very few published studies and interestingly enough, there are no published studies in the US, at least not that I am aware of, other than one obscure reprint of a study that was published in the Indian Journal of Dermatology that was reprinted online, by the Dermatology department of the University of California. This study substantiated the effects of taking zinc and its related effects on psoriasis, including some of what is in this book. I suppose if there were more published reports like the one by the Indian doctor who wrote the report, we would all have been taking it long ago and sending "Hope You're Doing Well" cards to our dermatologists, instead of checks. I have not seen my dermatologist since a few months after I became clear, just to show him, and have never seen any other dermatologist since then. That was over 30 years ago. What I had been told by my friend was an observation and theory that appears to be, at least by my experience, very true.

The reason I was told that zinc should provide skin improvement is that it is one of the more prominent minerals in your body and is required for normal skin development, growth and regeneration. It also is required for your immune system to work properly. It is the second most prominent trace mineral that is found in the body. Zinc is needed for the to help the body's autoimmune system and to maintain proper metabolism. Zinc is also needed to assist in wound healing and for the senses of smell and taste. Hmmm. It's almost common knowledge in the medical community. Anyway, it made sense to me at the time and still does today.

Zinc is the second most prominent trace mineral in the body, next only to iron. What is a bit unusual about zinc is that, unlike most of the other minerals needed by the body, zinc is not stored in our body. Most, if not all of the other minerals are. What this means is that you must constantly make sure that you have an adequate intake of zinc for your body to function at its optimum level and to maintain normal skin. Hmmm again. Makes sense to me.

One very interesting thing that I found was that the adrenal glands in your body normally produce cortisone and one of the things that occurs is that cortisone will tend to deplete the level of zinc in your system. This is also the case with virtually all the biologics that are now out. When the level of zinc is depleted in your system, it can only be surmised that normal skin development becomes rather abnormal. What does that sound like? Now, according to what I was told, we psoriasis sufferers most likely have abnormally low levels of zinc in our system, to begin with. At this point, I am totally convinced that that is the case. I was also told that when you are under stress, your body produces cortisone in greater amounts, further depleting the levels of zinc in your system. At this point I must add that, to my knowledge, there are no formal studies that have ever been conducted to substantiate this theory. These were the observations of my friend and something that made a lot of sense to me.

This theory in regards to the effects of cortisone on zinc levels in the body, which by my experience, appears to be true. It may just provide some explanation as to why cortisone derivative, topical medications work for some time, only to stop working completely and instead cause flare-ups that can be worse than the original condition. These topical steroids treat the symptom but, at the same time, may actually further deplete the levels of zinc in your system over a certain period of time. This is primarily due to what is known as transdermal absorption, where your body actually absorbs the cortisone that is in a particular treatment. I was one of those who, like a lot of you, used different topicals at the same time, hopefully to somehow increase the chances of finding something that worked for me. Unfortunately, it did nothing but add to my misery.

With biologics, they suppress the immune system and increase the risk of certain infections. People who take biologics are more likely to get infections such as upper respiratory infections, pneumonia, urinary tract infections, and skin infections, among other opportunistic infections. Because biologics change the way your immune system works, they also pose some serious peripheral health risks. It is likely why those who chose to use biologics very often switch from one to the other, and so on, and continue on a never-ending process with again, no substantial long lasting results. I've heard in some of the internet support groups of some even using different types of medications at the same time, just like I used to. You may be thinking that it makes absolutely no sense, other than since we are all so desperate to find something that works, we'll try just about anything. Some people taking biologics may have a higher risk for diseases such as tuberculosis and hepatitis. Others may have a higher risk for certain types of cancer.

Ok, so cortisone represses the zinc levels in your body and biologics suppress your immune system. It is generally recognized that psoriasis is an auto-immune issue. Why in the world would anyone prescribe something that reduces the mineral known to be required for normal skin and prescribe something that suppresses your immune system? It just doesn't make any sense to me whatsoever. In hindsight what it does is somewhat explain why they tend to only work for a while. What are in these medications that are supposed to help us? Now, as I've said before, I'm not a physician, nor do I have any medical background or training but, having lived with this condition for over 50 years and researching this affliction for more than half of my life, these questions about topical steroids and biologics are questions that I've never been able to fully answer. I have just been able to develop, what I would consider, very sound theories about what works, what doesn't, and probably why they don't work.

These prescription medications seem similar to a cleaning fluid used to remove spots or stains. You must be very careful to use the right amount. If you pay too much attention to the stain and use the slightest bit too much, you would be most likely to remove the stain, only to find out later that the stained fabric is now damaged even more than it was before.

There have been several studies, by various groups, in reference to the effects of zinc on the system. None have drawn any definite conclusions and seem to often conflict in some of their observations. None of the conclusions of any of these reports, that I have found, have determined any definite physical side effects of large amounts of zinc in the system, only digestive upset and possible diarrhea. Those possible side effects are not even remotely close to the known side effects of the prescription medications that we have been on. I mention this because the amount of zinc that is in what is now Psorclear, that I take each day, is well above what is referred to as the "recommended daily amount" for the average individual. What appears, at least to me, to be very odd is that this "recommended daily amount" does not seem to take into account body weight and the varying body metabolisms, related to different body weights. I am what I would consider average size for a man (6'1" / 200 pounds) and my so-called recommended dosage is the same as for someone who is less than half my weight.

The side effects that are described in these studies about zinc use the word “toxic”. That terminology, in itself, is wrong. What is referred to as toxic, when it relates to zinc/ion compounds that are formulated as dietary mineral supplements is incorrect and is actually a fallacy and not toxic at all. Something physically toxic is poisonous and can kill you. The only effects from a zinc dietary compound, such as Psorclear, are digestive discomfort and possible diarrhea, which I would definitely not call a physically toxic effect. It will just aggravate your digestive tract, which could happen due to taking excessive amounts of zinc. Psorclear, as you will see later, has been formulated to help reduce and/or eliminate those possible side effects from occurring.

It is important to note that zinc poisoning or, true toxicity, comes from ingesting or inhaling alloys or compounds (such as zinc chloride or zinc dithiophosphate) used for zinc plating or additives to items such as oil. Something toxic can kill you, like methotrexate. What methotrexate actually does do and why it's used for cancer chemotherapy and to treat psoriasis, as I said in the earlier Chapter, it drastically inhibits the reproduction of rapidly reproducing cells. However, it is non-discriminatory and attacks all of the rapidly reproducing cells in your body. Methotrexate, both in tablet form or injected, is also known to have substantial unpleasant and potentially dangerous side effects, as do most of the other prescription medications that are currently available.

My reason for shedding light on this matter may not be relevant for any other reason than to suggest that no one seems to know what vitamins and minerals really do for what, or so it seems. Ask a physician and most will say they don't do much of anything. Ask a homeopathic doctor or nutritionist and they will say it has everything to do with everything. To give credit where credit is due, there are some vitamins and minerals that are known to have specific effects on the body but, nothing is fully known. No one seems to have spent any substantial time studying the full effects of large amounts of vitamins and minerals on a body's system. Quite the contrary, it is much easier to go into a store and find mega-dose, multi-vitamin tablets, than it is to find half dosages. It has been proven to me, at least through my experience as a psoriasis sufferer that the zinc level in one's body does make a big difference based on what I have seen happen to my skin. As I have mentioned before, there is the possibility that the zinc level in a person with psoriasis may be depleted, to begin with. Now, compounding that with the changing of body weight and metabolism, as well as stress, that may deplete zinc levels even further, just may explain why people come down with psoriasis at different times in their lives.

One thing that I have found out since I've been taking what is now Psorclear, is some of the topicals that are solely for reducing scaling work quite well, and the results are much more prolonged. I will, from time to time, use a topical. The amount I use is minute, in comparison to what I used to use, once upon a time. To give you an idea of how much I use now, I have a 15gr. tube of fluocinonide .05% gel that I purchased in 2008, 13 years ago, and still have about half of the tube left. It undoubtedly expired a very long time ago but, I still keep it around as my security blanket and haven't needed it at all for a very long time now. There was a time back in the day, when I would use a 120gr. tube in a week. I cannot tell you how incredibly happy I am now. The amount of time I used to spend, on a day-to-day basis, just to barely make it through the day compared to what I do today, if anything, was and is literally life changing.

Now, I suppose you're wondering why I'm still using topical medications if this works so well. That's simple. Psorclear is still just a treatment that I use, even though it is the most effective one I've ever used. However, as I will explain in more detail later on, the area of my body that has always been the hardest to control has been my scalp. While the effect on my body, arms, legs and fingernails has been amazing since I started taking it, my scalp psoriasis has greatly improved but, it still exists be it as minor as it is. However, I still find it very helpful to use only shampoos with salicylic acid in them and not coal tar. I use this to help eliminate any redness at my hairline and any very small spots that may crop up in my scalp. It is the only type of shampoo that I use.

Now, this is only my personal opinion. Based on how Psorclear has worked for me but, it only seems logical that this treatment just may have a positive effect on psoriatic arthritis too. Since I don't have that affliction, this is only a supposition on my part. I have been told by those who have psoriatic arthritis that Psorclear does help with the pain and movement. That too makes total sense, especially since it has been clinically proven in studies that those who suffer from the various forms of arthritis, including psoriatic arthritis have a significant zinc serum deficiency. Overall, in my experience from hearing from others who have used Psorclear, the feedback has been amazing and I hope my words are encouraging enough for you to give it a try.

What is interesting is that a lot of you will go to rheumatologists for treatments that are very often expensive, again with no lasting results. Just as is the case with dermatologists who suffer from psoriasis and know what it's like to deal with it, there are about 4,997 practicing rheumatologists in the United States today. Of that number, only about 100 most likely are suffering from psoriasis. Of that number only about 20 of them probably suffer from psoriatic arthritis, based on the known odds and numbers. Ok, we again have a situation where we (thank

God not me) are being treated by someone who has just studied, observed and practiced on those of us who are willing to be their guinea pigs. No wonder we're all so confused about what's right, what's wrong and, more importantly, what really works. We Psoriasis sufferers are always so desperate to try whatever we can find to help us to be just normal like other people. We continually go to doctor after doctor, hoping to find something or someone who can really help. All we get are prescription products and treatments from medical practitioners and corporations who may or may not have our best interest at heart.

I've written this book to tell you as much as I possibly can about my journey, what I discovered and of how nothing worked for me, until something did. That something is now Psorclear™.

4

More Good Stuff

Now, this is what I did to get my psoriasis under control and continue to do till this day.

Earlier in the book I told you that I now take Psorclear, which is nothing more than the brand name for a common zinc/copper compound that has been formulated especially for effective treatment of psoriasis and eczema, as well as other related skin conditions. Back in the beginning, I started to take regular zinc tablets, a mineral easily found over the counter, without a prescription. It can be purchased in various quantities, usually from 50 to 250 tablets per bottle. Each tablet is either 50 or 100 mg.(milligrams) in dosage, so I started using the 100mg ones. A 50 mg tablet is supposedly 333% of the recommended daily amount of zinc for a normal person. Again, there is no adjustment in recommended daily amount based on a person's weight, which seems a bit odd. It seems to me to be a case of one size fits all and that just isn't true.

During my worst case of psoriasis, I took two tablets per day, what I thought was the equivalent of 200 mg of zinc per day. It worked but, only slightly. I decided to increase the dosage to four tablets per day. That happened to work best for my weight, 200 lbs. at that time. That was one tablet per each 50 lbs. of body weight. For those of you on the metric system, it amounts to one tablet per 23 kg of body weight. In my research, I found that a 100 mg. tablet of zinc consisted of 23% elemental zinc. Because of the serious stomach upset from these tablets, I had to split the dosage. I took two tablets each morning and two each night before bed. At the time, I was not educated about zinc but, I learned and learned a lot. I never increased my dosage from 4 a day to see if there was any additional or faster clearing of the psoriasis. I was so pleased with the effect from using the amount I was using, I did not feel the need, nor did I have the desire. I figured that what I was taking was enough and I don't think that my stomach could have handled any more. About 30 years ago, I managed to reach the point where my skin was almost completely clear, about 99% clear. Needless to say, at that time I did not feel the need to experiment with increased dosages. I have been virtually totally clear since then, with almost none to ever return, except for a very small unrecognizable spot upon occasion.

I started by taking 200 mg (two 100 mg. tablets) per day, based on what my friend had suggested and that is exactly what I did. I found out, after about the first couple weeks, that the infernal itching that had plagued me for years began to slightly subside. That in itself was a God send. I used to tell people who asked me what the itching was like, that it was as if you were running naked through the Amazon rain forest, 15 minutes after the rain had stopped and the mosquitos came out.

I then increased the dosage to see if it worked better. I began taking 200 mg each morning and 200 mg each night, and it did work better, as I had suspected. This accelerated the effects and, within the next two weeks, I noticed that the heat generated on the lesions began to decrease steadily. The next few weeks, the redness began to gradually disappear, as the scales were lessening on the smaller spots on my body. The horrendous itching was nearly gone. The scale on the larger areas and most of the areas were very large, became lighter and lighter. The small patches of redness and scale were gradually disappearing by the end of the first month. I was now noticing that the small spots and patches were disappearing, almost on a daily basis.

After the third month, just about all the redness and scale had disappeared. There were still some areas of my body that were and still are affected. However, I was the only one who knew that these spots still existed. The minor flare-ups that did occur, at least in my case, were directly related to certain activities, which I will explain later. In the cold, dry winter of Chicago, where I live, flare-ups occur more frequently. Now though, they are not noticeable to the average person as anything more than a minor rash or a normal skin blemish.

By the end of the third month, my fingernails also began to go back to being normal. The pitting even began to disappear. Today, all the pitting has gone and has never returned. My fingernails and toenails had always been the cause of embarrassment for me because I could not hide them and the deformation was grotesque. Once, while on a cruise, my wife at that time, had insisted I get a manicure. I had never had one and she actually thought that it might help. Her intention was just another one of those thoughtful yet, meaningless treatment suggestions. Well, after working on my nails for quite some time, the manicurist just looked at me and said, "I'm sorry, there's nothing I can do". That's how bad they were for all those years. Now, nobody notices them because they're normal.

I never thought I would be able to stop vacuuming the bed every day, which is what I had to do for so many years. I could barely remember a day I did not have to do it. I moved into a new condominium about two years after I'd been on the zinc tablets and, to this day, I haven't been able to find my dust buster. I haven't missed it, nor have I needed it for anything.

The psoriasis in my scalp had lessened to the point that there are only very rare small spots that show up occasionally. I have not had complete success with my scalp as I have had with the rest of my body. I suspect that this is the same reason that scalp psoriasis and eczema are the hardest to control. There is only a skin covering to the top portion of the skull and no muscle tissue. There are no major blood vessels in the skin, just small capillaries. The normal blood flow that is in the rest of the body is just not there in the scalp. Not only does that make the skin more susceptible to having either psoriasis or eczema but, also makes it more difficult for an adequate amount of the minerals needed for normal skin growth and regeneration to get to it. My scalp psoriasis however, is greatly improved from what it has been like for years. Like with the other parts of my body, now only I know I have psoriasis, and no longer do I look like I have a massive amount of dandruff. It has all gone from my shoulders. My scalp used to feel as if a helmet was glued to my head.

The scales are now incredibly minor, in comparison, and virtually gone. The scalp itching has stopped completely and there is virtually no flaking. It used to be so bad that I couldn't wear dark-colored clothes because of the excessive flaking. That is not the case now, as I'm now even wearing black shirts.

It had actually reached the point that I had lost quite a bit of hair and even began to develop a bald spot because of it. Now, for the most part (I am 72), all my hair has returned, except for the hair that most old guys usually lose. Later I will explain what I do with my scalp and the other spots that have flared up slightly, from time to time, as well as why these minor flare-ups are more prevalent on that part of my body.

I now take a maintenance dosage of what has come to be Psorclear, one-half of what I used to take when I was first fighting this. I take two capsules per day, usually first thing in the morning. I'm, however, only human and do sometimes forget, especially on the weekends. When I skip a number of days, usually a few days straight, is when I notice very minor flare-ups. Once I get back to the normal dosage that I take, these flare-ups subside. When I do forget, I don't double the dosage the next time, so I do not know if doing so would have an effect on minimizing the occasional minor flare-ups. Again, the flare-ups are so minor that it doesn't bother me at all, so I personally never found the need to see if that would help. Thankfully, I’ve been almost totally clear ever since then and still am, for almost 30 years now.

I did stop taking the zinc tablets that I was taking at that time, back when my psoriasis first cleared up. I did this on purpose. I wanted to find out two things:

1) If I could stop and the psoriasis would never return and,

2) To find out if it did come back, would it come back worse than before, as it always did with the other medications.

What I found was that it did come back, although it did take longer than ever before and when it did, it was not nearly as bad as it was before. Once I started taking the tablets again, it actually cleared up faster than before. I would suspect that if I stopped taking it too soon and let the redness and scaling return as it was before, I would probably need to start all over. It would probably take about the same amount of time as it originally did for it to come back under control.

I also cut the dosage once, right after the psoriasis had cleared up, to see if a lower dosage would maintain the clearing effect. It didn't. After some time, it slowly started to come back. I went back to taking the dosage of zinc that I had been taking regularly. But again, like before, it cleared up at a faster rate. At that point, I figured that I should keep taking the amount that I had been taking for some extended period of time after my skin was clear. I continued to take it regularly for the next five years before I again reduced it to a lower maintenance dosage. Since I was so pleased with the results, I didn’t keep experimenting to see if I could go to a maintenance dosage sooner. That may be possible but, I didn't want to take another step back to find out. It was about that time that I had contacted a manufacturer to see if they would formulate Psorclear. It was, by far, much better on my stomach and it worked and still does to this day. To this day I take two capsules a day and will continue to do so, until someone finally finds a permanent cure. I'm not holding out too much hope and I would recommend you do the same.

Now that I've told you what I did, still do, and how it has positively affected my psoriasis, I do have to take the time to tell you about the only adverse side effect that I've found and what I do to combat it. There's actually only one adverse effect that I've found over the period of time when I had been taking the common zinc tablets and it has to do more with how I took them and when. That side effect did not occur once, when I started taking the newly formulated Psorclear. I do consider it to be a virtually non-existent side effect when I compare it to the potentially very serious side effects that are known to possibly occur with some of the other medications that I've used in the past.

The one adverse side effect of taking large doses of zinc tablets that I discovered was that, when I took them on an empty stomach, it did seriously upset it. Unfortunately, I am one of those who does not like to eat first thing in the morning or late at night, so I lived with it for the most part. It always happened when I would take them on an empty stomach and I wasn't quite sure why. There were times when I would almost immediately throw up. Being bull-headed as I am, admittedly, I figured that, since I had just thrown up there couldn't be anything left so, I would take them again. I was bound and determined to find out if this would work, even if I had to withstand the bad side effects.

As you will find out later, I did eventually find out why that happened. I just dealt with it whenever it did happen. I found, at the time, that taking the zinc tablets with food did help in easing my upset stomach. However, even the upsetting effect from taking the tablets was nowhere near as serious as the nauseating effect that psoralens or, some of the other oral prescriptions had on me, not to mention that the possible side effects from some of the prescription drugs was very scary.

There are times when I had to eat something in the morning and, when I did, the upsetting feeling subsided. Back when I was taking zinc tablets and was originally fighting this affliction, at times, my stomach became too upset to allow me to sleep. That was when I took the tablets before bed on an empty stomach. I found that, when I took them in the evening, if I ate even just some ice cream or yogurt before I went to bed, it had the same soothing effect and the feeling subsided.

Once Psorclear was formulated, I took four capsules a day and I was able to take them all at one time. Only on very rare occasions, would it cause an uncomfortable feeling but, and I stress this, only on an empty stomach. Anything I ate did eliminate the extremely uncomfortable side effects and all the agony, indigestion that I was experiencing. What was, back then, incredible discomfort was now gone. That only confirmed, even more, what I had thought about the fillers in the regular zinc tables being the main cause of my problem with taking them.

Before I leave this chapter, there is one other side effect (a good one) that I've noticed since I've been taking the zinc tablets and now what is Psorclear. I don't seem to get common colds any more. I have not had one in years! Funny thing, Huh?

5

The Story of Psorclear

When I was using regular zinc tablets, some would make me drastically sick and some wouldn't. I really didn't figure out what caused this until I started reading their labels to see what the "inactive ingredients" were that were used as fillers to make these tablets. They were different for every manufacturer. Some even had stuff in them that are known to be allergens, which may cause allergic reactions for some people. Thank God I don't have any allergies and never have had any. I do empathize with those who do. Having psoriasis is bad enough for me. That's when I realized that it wasn't necessarily the zinc that was making me sick. It was what is used as fillers.

I then started doing research on what zinc/ion compounds consisted of, which were used to create the tablets. There's zinc gluconate, zinc picolinate, zinc sulphate and several other compounds that aren't normally used to create a zinc dietary supplement. Zinc sulphate didn't work at all and I found that this was stated in several studies. Zinc gluconate seemed to work best for me.

I had to take quite a bit for it to work and I found out, through my research that in a 100 mg. tablet of both zinc gluconate and zinc picolinate, there was only about 23-24% elemental zinc. In some there was even less, about half that amount. The rest were the binding agents used to form the compound, not to mention the fillers used to form the tablets. That pretty much explained it to me. I realized that since each tablet only had about 23-24 mg. of elemental zinc, I figured that if I had a compound formulated that consisted of about 25mg. of elemental zinc and add a non-allergenic filler, that wouldn't make me sick. It would be substantially beneficial in reducing the bad side effects that I had experienced taking the amount of zinc tablets that I needed to take to achieve any meaningful results. It was formulated with only vegetable cellulose as a filler and it worked! The bad side effect that was a regular occurrence was gone!

As mentioned earlier, there are published studies about excessive amounts of zinc being, so called, toxic. Some of those studies state that 250 mg. per day is the highest recommended intake. Some say 300 mg. and some even say that up to 1,000 mg. per day is acceptable. The FDA states that the recommended daily requirement is 15 mg. No one knows for sure, it seems, or at least there is no common agreement. Again, the FDA makes no adjustment in this recommendation for body size.

Like I've said, Psorclear™ is nothing more than a brand name for a zinc/ion compound that has been specially formulated and is water-soluble. What this means is that whatever amount of zinc that you take that your body doesn't need is expelled from your body. If that is the case, and I believe from my research that it is, then the possibility of zinc toxicity as it relates to mineral supplements seems, at least to me, to be a total fallacy. For some strange reason, there have never been many detailed studies conducted on exactly what happens when you take what is considered to be excessive amounts of zinc, except for the known digestive side effects. There are just these "toxicity" warnings that seem to be invalid. The only studies that I have found relating to any substantial benefits of taking, what is considered to be, large amounts of zinc are the foreign studies that I have found, related to psoriasis and other skin afflictions.

It just doesn't make any sense to me to call digestive discomfort toxic. It's just very uncomfortable. Many of these studies seem to muddle up the different types of zinc compounds, probably being the reason to use the term toxic. Some definitely are toxic but, those are not the zinc/ion compounds used to formulate dietary supplements. Maybe there's a monetary reason for the lack of such studies and purposeful use of the word “toxic”. That’s just my opinion, for what it’s worth.

Psorclear has been formulated to substantially reduce and, in most cases, totally eliminate the possibility of experiencing any of the known side effects of digestive upset and possible diarrhea. I’m sure some of you will still experience them, as I have. However, when it does occur it is much milder and is on much rarer frequency than when I was taking regular zinc tablets. Those side effects pale in comparison to the benefit that I have had in clearing my psoriasis.

Psorclear has been specifically formulated as a zinc/copper compound. The reason for this combination is that it is known that zinc can cause depletion of copper in one’s body. Copper depletion is not a good thing. Even doctors, unless you’re a hematologist, have little to no idea of the critically essential importance that copper has in the body. It is used to aid the absorption of other minerals, such as zinc and iron, and is also the primary nutrient for baby blood cells. Your bone marrow manufactures blood cells but, to have them reach puberty and be useful for your body, they need copper. Without it, they die and you end up depleting the blood that your body has. Blood cells in your body constantly die and are replaced by new ones. Unfortunately, I found this out the hard way by suffering from a copper deficiency once myself.

It was caused by other medical issues that I experienced, not from taking too much zinc. That's when I learned what purpose copper serves in your body. When I was first admitted to the hospital, they gave me 5 pints of blood transfusions. I had used up half of my blood and had become unbelievably weak. I actually ended up having regular copper transfusions for almost a year after my discharge from the hospital. At first twice a week, then once a week. It is for those very important reasons that copper was added to the Psorclear compound.

Psorclear has also been formulated to eliminate any of the fillers that had caused me such discomfort. It is also highly recommended that Psorclear be taken with food, in order to help further reduce the possibility of those unwanted side effects from occurring. There are no allergenic fillers in Psorclear. The only filler that is used is vegetable cellulose. Vegetable cellulose is a non-digestible plant fiber and our body needs non-digestible vegetable fiber, which is available in some of our food. That's why people eat bran flakes and other fibrous foods. Fiber is also needed for the body to function properly and aid digestion.

It is non-allergenic, wheat and gluten free. Psorclear contains none of the other following allergens: yeast, soy protein, milk or dairy products, corn, sodium, sugar, starch, artificial coloring, preservatives, flavoring, lactose, nuts or nut by-products, or caffeine. Psorclear is manufactured in the US, in Oklahoma to be exact. It is manufactured using FDA approved minerals and additives. It's made using GMP (Good Manufacturing Practice) guidelines that are set by the FDA.

Psorclear was also formulated in capsule form to allow you to break the capsule apart and mix the contents with food or drinks. This is to accommodate those who have difficulty swallowing hard pills and also as another way to help eliminate the possible side effects. Every precaution has been taken by the manufacturer to make sure that the unwanted side effects, if any, that I experienced from taking regular zinc tablets have been, to the best possible degree, eliminated.

Being a common mineral supplement, Psorclear doesn’t interact with other drugs or medical conditions, like a lot of the prescription medications that are out there. Every bad experience that I had with regular zinc tablets was either drastically reduced or eliminated in the formulation of Psorclear. I have survived cancer, a serious blood disorder, a heart attack, a serious stomach disorder and a stroke. I take ten different medications each day and Psorclear hasn’t interfered with any of those medications, nor has it created any adverse physical conditions. Needless to say, I know this because I am monitored and tested on a regular basis by my doctors and have been for years now. Nothing as such has ever been found.

The first thing that most notice, when you do start taking Psorclear, is that the itching will begin to subside, usually within a couple weeks. Soon, the redness and scaling will begin to diminish. It can take 2-3 months before you notice substantial clearing, depending on how bad your condition is. It can take up to 4 months to see results, depending on how much zinc deficiency you may have and your BMI (body mass index). Some do see substantial results sooner, usually those who suffer from minor cases of psoriasis or those with eczema. I suspect, in the case of psoriasis, that is because the zinc level in their body hasn't depleted to the point that it would take a lot of time to replenish it.

As stated before, the dosage that I used and what seems to have the greatest success is one capsule per each 50 lbs. (23 kg.) of body weight taken daily. Should you take less, there is a very good chance that you will see little to no results. It is not a quick fix by any stretch of the imagination. Even most prescription medications are not. It is not a drug. It's a mineral supplement that replenishes the minerals that have been clinically proven to be needed for health skin and to be helpful to those with psoriasis. It takes time for it to have an effect, only after your body has built up enough to compensate for your mineral deficiency.

Most who do not experience relief from using Psorclear are those who:

1). Do not take it for a long enough period of time to see adequate results.

2). Do not take the dosage of one capsule per each 50 lbs. (23 kg.) of body weight daily.

3). Stop taking it as soon as they see results and experience their psoriasis reoccurring, which it will.

4). Have other medical pre-existing conditions that may work to aggravate their psoriasis and/or may inhibit their ability to absorb the minerals at an adequate level to experience relief.

There are a lot of people who seem to think Psorclear is a miracle drug. Well, it's not. It's just a common mineral supplement that works.

With scalp and nail psoriasis, it does take much longer and with scalp psoriasis, it takes additional special care to bring it under control. Scalp and nail psoriasis are the two most difficult types to deal with and treat. Psorclear works on both. With scalp psoriasis, it is very important that you only use mild shampoos. As I found out through experimentation, what seems to work best for me are shampoos that have only salicylic acid in them, not coal tar or salicylic acid/coal tar combinations. Those were the least irritating and seem to be the most helpful.

Psoriasis, as you well know, is open sores due to the incredibly fast skin reproduction. I would highly suggest not using any hair conditioners at all. Most of the commercial shampoos and conditioners that are on the market, including the dandruff shampoos with zinc in them for dandruff sufferers, will irritate your psoriasis, aggravate your scalp and not help with the relief. While a lot of them are supposed to be good for your hair, they can be extremely devastating to the scalp of someone with scalp psoriasis, which I have personally found to be true. Almost all of the shampoos and conditioners that are on the market have chemicals in them that seriously aggravate scalp psoriasis. Whenever I used any regular shampoo, my scalp psoriasis would start to reappear noticeably.

The primary reason that it takes longer for substantial clearing in your scalp is that it does not have the blood flow that the rest of your body has, as I mentioned in the earlier chapter. This is because it is just a layer of skin with no muscle tissue. With fingernail and toenail psoriasis, it will take some time for them to grow back out. What you will notice first is that the pitting in your nails will begin to disappear and the discoloration below your nails will begin to come back to, what used to be, normal. From there, after a bit of time, your nails will return to normal, as mine have done.

You might be asking yourself, is it safe for kids? The answer is yes, but with adult supervision. Psorclear is in capsule form and the effective dosage, as I have found, is one capsule for every 50 lbs. (23 kg.) of a person's body weight. For this reason, it is relatively impractical to give it to anyone under that weight, like a child under the age of about 6. It would be possible to empty the capsule contents and try to measure out a smaller amount but, that would be somewhat impractical. It is, however, based on the weight of a person, not their age.

Regarding any skin discoloration that may occur once the scale and redness is gone, it will eventually disappear. It just takes time for what is now normal skin to normally regenerate. That time will undoubtedly vary from person to person. For me, it took about one year. As of writing the initial booklet, all the discolored spots that were where I did have it and I had a lot, were all gone and I have never had anything else but normal-looking skin ever since. That was almost 30 years ago. I now wear both shorts and short sleeve shirts in the summer almost daily. I now go swimming too.

As for your hair growing back after you've been able to stop picking at your scalp, which you will eventually stop doing, yes, your hair will eventually grow back once all the redness and scales are gone. That is if you had a full head of hair prior to contracting scalp psoriasis. If you are prone to baldness, your head will return to what was normal for you and, like with the rest of your body, the skin discoloration will eventually totally disappear.

Now you're probably asking yourself if it worked so well, why did it take so long for this to come out to the general public? That's a difficult question to answer. Once I found it worked so well, I eventually didn't even consider myself as actually having psoriasis. My condition became so minuscule to me that it became a non-issue. At the time, I did write the other booklet and had self-published it but, due to other occupational responsibilities that were mounting, I stopped putting the book out. I figured that, once I retired, I'd rewrite the book and see about getting it published. Well, I never retired and still haven't. People like me just don't. We don't know how.

Then I started seeing all the advertising come out for all the "new stuff" that, for the most part, was just like what I used and only worked for a while. I've seen story after story in internet support groups from people who have tried one after another of the new biologics, all with no good results. As much as I don't want to, I'll give you my thoughts on internet support groups later. Back to these commercials. They all got me incredibly irritated, as they have probably done to those of you who, like me, have suffered for countless years. All those commercials are for the "newbies", the ones who have just contracted psoriasis or, have just had it for a short period of time, not 20-30 years or more.

I then contacted the company that formulated it for me from what was in my original booklet and asked them if they'd bottle it and put it out for general consumption. The answer was yes and Psorclear™ became something more than my own personal remedy. That finally motivated me to rewrite this book and tell my story. I am including all the information I researched and experienced after almost 30 years of being totally clear. At the same time, my story just might be of some help to promote Psorclear and help all of you who have hoped for some help that really works.

As I stated above, it has been reported that Psorclear does not work for everyone, which is why I went through the reasons it may not. It works wonderfully for me and has for many, many years now. It has also worked for many others who have tried it. It just might be worth a try for you.

Should you wish to try Psorclear, it is now available at Amazon US, Amazon Australia, Amazon Singapore and soon, from what I understand from the manufacturer, at Amazon Mexico. It is also available on Walmart online, eBay, Wish and on the Psorclear.com website. Hopefully soon it will be in retail stores. There is a lot of other good information on Psorclear's website and it just might be worth checking it out. There's a lot of actual reviews by those who have found Psorclear to work for them, as well as answers to a lot of other questions that you may have, after reading this book.

6

Now, What You Don't Want to Hear.

I'm not quite sure why this hasn't been formulated and promoted by the medical community as an inexpensive, effective and consistent means of treating both psoriasis and eczema. I can only speculate. It has been reported in some clinical studies that zinc is necessary for your body and is incredibly important for your normal skin growth and its regeneration. This is common knowledge within the medical community but not spoken about, as I mentioned before. Is it possible that more money is made by merely treating the outward symptoms than by treating the cause? The reason this hasn't been formulated and marketed to psoriasis and eczema sufferers, before now, is as good your guess as mine. As I've said earlier in the book, it has now been almost 30 years since I last saw a dermatologist or any other doctor for my psoriasis. Why in the world would my dermatologist tell me to use something that would work and risk losing a regular customer (oops, sorry…patient)? This may be an issue of not wanting to "bite the hand that feeds you", so to speak.

It also doesn't take into account the drug companies making fortunes selling prescription medication which only treat the external symptoms, if it does anything and does not treat the cause. They too have no reason to bite the hands that feed them either.

There are, to my knowledge at this time, over 224 prescription medications for psoriasis, all of which only treat the visible symptoms and not the cause. They come in the form of pills, ointments, creams and injectable medications. Some of the possible side effects can be devastating, even causing death. There are probably thousands of OTC (over the counter) creams and ointments that will only help mask the itching and redness and don't address the underlying cause. They are all, both OTC and prescription medications, temporary at best. We know this from what we've all been through, going from one treatment to the next and then to the next, not knowing if it is ever going to end, we're always hoping that someday, there will be something that will work. With prescription medications, they will only work until your body builds up a certain resistance to it. When it does, flare-ups are most likely to occur which are worse than when you first started taking the medication. This is primarily true for topical steroids, resulting in the condition called TSW (Topical Steroid Withdrawal), where your body absorbs the steroids that are in the topical medications. Topical steroids can also interact with different types, if you happen to be using more than one at the same time. This can either cancel out its effect or, in turn, make the situation you are dealing with, at the time, even worse. I'm not an expert, as I have said before but, there is a website where you can go to read more about TSW, such as its causes and effects. They seem to have covered the Topical Steroid Withdrawal Syndrome fairly well. The website is https://Itsan.org.

What is totally amazing to me and somewhat disturbing is the success rates of many of these popular prescription medications. They are rated based on what is called "SR", Success Rate, which is a percentage of clarity after 4 months of treatment. The SR for these new "wonder drugs" varies from 32-85%. I guess they feel that partially clear is good enough. Maybe it's good enough for them but, we want to be normal, so we can get back to the life we used to know, the life we once lived. Good enough is what we've dealt with ever since we came down with this and good enough isn't what we want. Again, these medications are most likely developed by individuals and groups who have not personally experienced this condition and do not know how demoralizing the thought of merely "something is better than nothing" really feels like. We've heard this all our lives and never felt that wearing a short sleeve shirt with a long pair of pants on a hot day was much consolation. There isn't a single one of us who would not have sold our sole for a pair of shorts or, maybe even a swimming suit. If we have toenail psoriasis, we can't even wear a pair of sandals. I didn't do any of that for over 20 years, and I lived every single day, hoping that someday, something would work. Those days are now past me, after what became Psorclear was suggested to me.

The cost of most of the prescription medications that are available, especially the biologics, are astronomical and only affordable if you have either great insurance or, if you qualify for low-income assistance. In either case, it is very likely that eventually the insurer will either reduce the amount of payment or, discontinue it altogether.

I believe a cure will undoubtedly eventually be found and, it will most likely be found by some researcher who has the condition. When? Your guess is as good as mine. There are 16 diseases that, at one time, were considered incurable. However, since then they have been either eradicated globally or, have been eliminated regionally. Psoriasis and eczema may very well someday be two more conditions that may join that group and no longer torment us for our entire lives.

Now for my least favorite part of this book and the topic on which I do only admittedly, have second hand knowledge. My editors asked that I expound on the social media aspect of having to deal with this disease but, since I now consider myself to be virtually clear of psoriasis and have been for so long, I never did participate in any conversations with anyone in those support groups. All I can really write about are my mere observations. On rare occasion, in the past, I have created some simple posts telling people how Psorclear helped change my life. However, I have stopped doing that. Most of the time, when I did post, the only responses would be from others who have "The Cure". Occasionally I would get a "Thumbs Up" or two but, never any real conversation about my postings. I suspect I was put in the same category as those who had "The Cure," even though after reading this much of this book, you have probably realized that is not the case. What never ceases to amaze me is that, us being one of the most skeptical groups of people on earth, why so many gravitate to those “half baked” remedies, treatments and supposed “Cures”? To me it is a case of the blind leading the blind and hoping to get some valuable advice from those who don’t really know. “Dr. Google” isn’t really any help either. You can get several different answers to the same question. Again, it is a lot of conflicting information that is of little or no help at all. You just get what others think you should know or, want you to know. I’ve read some questions and answers in those support groups that were so far out in left field that it was almost mind boggling. I guess, just like I did when I suffered from it, we are always looking hopefully for something that finally works, something that will finally take us out of our misery. That is why I found someone who would create Psorclear, because it worked so well for me. Admittedly, the company does run ads on social media platforms but, they aren’t meant to be anything other than an advertisement to promote the product. They are not disguised as personal or medical advice, which is often the case in various support sites.

There are purported support sites that have been created by people for no other reason than to sell either their philosophy about the disease. They also promote the sale of some other product, that most likely won't work for long, if it works at all. It seems like the bulk of these types of sites are created in countries outside of the US. One of my favorite support sites (I say that tongue in cheek) is "Psoriasis-Eczyma can be cured". It's hard for me to understand how someone who can't even spell eczema could have a cure or, even a supposedly valid treatment for it. Maybe it's just me being incredibly skeptical. At least they spelled psoriasis correctly. Another one of my favorites is "Psoriasis Treatment Free for Life". This one seems to be full of posts telling you to contact them. Maybe it's just me again but, I doubt that they're offering free advice or that anything is really "free" as they so adamantly put it.

As I see it, there are advantages and disadvantages of social media and social media support groups. There's a bunch of them and everyone one who is on them has their own idea and opinion of what works and what does not. Most, as you have probably already found, are either half-baked, totally off base or, just someone's thoughts on what may work. Then there are those posting about doctors, usually in foreign countries, who have found "the cure". Most of those are absolutely ludicrous. They prey on those who have yet to either determine their condition, or have not yet understood that there is no cure. You can tell by the questions that some ask. It's sad. Some don't have any idea of what psoriasis or eczema is really about, much less the ramifications of having it. Some can't even spell psoriasis. There are a lot who depend on others for free advice. There is that saying that I mentioned back in Chapter One that "free advice is worth exactly what you pay for it"...nothing. That's exactly what you get.

Social media can be quite harsh on people too, especially those who have already developed a very low self-esteem from having either psoriasis or eczema. A lot of the posts and responses that I have seen are sad, some incredibly sad. In doing my research, I have monitored over

20 different support groups on various platforms. Most of the time they're either sad or, most times, a question or the answers are not the least bit helpful. It's just someone else putting in their "two cents".

It appears, from what I've seen that there are a lot of people who use social media and support groups, just to prop up their egos while not really providing any meaningful contribution. Thankfully I haven't seen many derogatory remarks or posts about me and/or Psorclear, like those that are common on the majority of the social media sites, as a whole. It seems that most of the moderators of these support group sites don't allow any type of demeaning remarks to be posted. What I do see are some incredibly off-beat posts. That's why I do the best I can to stay away from any of those sites, other than to see what's going on there.

The most memorable response that I have seen by anyone, regarding a suggested treatment for psoriasis, was the woman who posted this response and I quote, "Just eliminate your stress and swim in salt water". I guess for her, turning all the adverse things that happen to you in your life into mere inconsequential or meaningless events is easy. Oh Yeah? And, she must live on the coast of a coast state, because it's quite difficult to turn a normal, fresh-water swimming pool into a salt water one. Nor can we all afford to just pack up and move to a coastal beach area. So, if you're looking for good advice on how to treat your condition and if you like social media, go there and get more advice just like this. This is just one more reason why so many people are so confused about what to do to treat their psoriasis or eczema effectively.

In the first part of the book, I said that I would not say anything about the psychological trauma that I went through, since you know all about that. However, there is one very interesting and very sad thing that I have heard and I thought that it was worth relaying to you. It was a few years ago and was related to the psychological trauma that one can go through with both psoriasis and eczema. It was in a newspaper article that I read, not a comment in a support group. It was an article in the New York Daily

News on June 20, 2018. The story was about a young woman who lived in Hong Kong who had killed both her parents, then committed suicide. Her relatives told police that the reason she had killed them is because she blamed them both for her having eczema and for it ruining her life. She also took her own life because she just couldn't go on. That is, without a doubt, the saddest story that I have ever heard, in over 50 years of dealing with this affliction. I mention this only because I really wonder how many people go through such severe psychological trauma and they end up going to these internet support groups to hopefully get some help and guidance and what they end up getting is anything but that.

I wonder just how many of us there are who are so distraught that we do not know where to turn for help. Again, only those who know, know. I dealt with it, thanks to my incredibly warped sense of humor but, others aren't that lucky. For those of you who may be suffering, possibly not that badly but, bad enough for you, in my estimation it would be best to find some type of counselor who has had firsthand knowledge of the trauma it causes, not just someone who is a passive bystander and observer who offers off-handed advise. Those people just don't know what we're dealing with. I know that is an incredibly difficult person to find but, I see it as the only way anyone can find someone to relate to who can offer any meaningful advice. An internet support group just isn't the place to find that help. I've seen people post about their mental state, due to either psoriasis or eczema, and all they get are people telling them how sorry they are to hear about what they're going through. A simple "Sorry" just won't do it. Hopefully the information that is in this book can be your answer. It's really all any of us have ever wanted...an answer that really meant something. I found my answer and hopefully, after reading what's in here, you will too.

7

The Rest of the Story

As I have said throughout this book, Psorclear is NOT a cure, it's the most effective and consistent treatment I have ever known. It is also the safest, easiest and the least expensive solution that I've found of anything else out there. As I have said repeatedly in this book, there is no cure for psoriasis and eczema and I'm betting that no one ever will find one because the motivation is just not there.

Earlier I mentioned that I still have minor flare ups and that my scalp is not as clear as the rest of my body, though only noticeable to me. So, I should probably tell you what I do to keep my psoriasis under control, in both cases. I should also mention that I have, what might be called by some, an abundance of body hair. I personally think it's a normal amount for an adult male but, I do also tell people that I am living proof that man evolved from apes. Seriously though, I have noticed that it is the hairy areas that are the hardest to control and the most likely areas to flare up. Just in case you're wondering, those areas include the crotch area. The areas with little or no hair and I do have some of those, seem to stay the clearest and are the least prone to flare ups.

Like I said, the flare ups that I do have are almost totally insignificant, compared to anything I've had to deal with in the past regarding this affliction. What has happened is that I have become used to being "normal", now that it's been about thirty years since I've considered psoriasis a problem. When I do get minor flare ups, I take care of the areas. The only difference from before is that now it's just like just taking care of a minor irritation.

Sometimes the flare ups will just come and go all by themselves.

I still do occasionally use a topical steroid. However, I use it very, very sparingly and when I do use it, I use a much lesser than I used before because now it is much more effective and the results last much longer. I keep it on hand for two reasons. One is the force of habit. Even now, after all these years, I realize that I still have psoriasis and I just want to keep it around as a security blanket. Even I have a hard time realizing that this treatment has been and continues to be as effective as it is. It's almost funny to me how this affliction can have such a profound and lasting effect on my psyche. The other reason is that it works so much faster to eliminate the redness at my hairline, which is the hardest to control. I don't really need it but, I have just become impatient and want any minor spots that do show up...gone now! Now, when I do use it, I use it very, very sparingly. I put it on and rub it in.

Now for the scalp. As I said earlier, it is the hardest area to control, even harder than my fingernails. The thickest scale I have ever had was in my scalp, to the point of even losing hair. Now, the scale that does occur is very light and fairly easy to remove. Like I said before, I used to have to put topicals on my hair every night and wear a shower cap to bed. Back at that time, it didn't even help much, not to mention the extraordinary amounts I have had to use. The psoriasis in my scalp is now less than 1% of what it used to be. One thing that I have noticed is that in the summer, my scalp has even less scale than it does in the winters. This can only be due to the additional exposure to the sun. I'm guessing that having old guy thinning hair helps too.

Part of the reason that the scalp is the hardest area to control is because of all the stuff that we use on our hair to keep it in place or, however we want it, the right color and "soft and manageable". All of this stuff, no matter how mild that you may think that it may be, gets to the scalp and irritates the psoriasis or eczema! As I've said before, I use an inexpensive shampoo that has salicylic acid in it and does not have coal tar in it. The one I use is available at

Walgreens (their generic brand). To this day, I only use that type of shampoo to wash my hair. It's mild, doesn't have any offensive smell and works great. If I cannot get the generic shampoo, something similar is always available somewhere but, usually at a higher price. I have discovered that most, if not all regular shampoos on the market will definitely irritate my scalp and make the psoriasis noticeably worse, virtually overnight. After all, they've been developed for your hair and not your scalp. There are zinc shampoos on the market but they also have additives in them that are meant to help your hair but, don't do much to help your scalp, not to mention that they are expensive. They're primarily for those who suffer from dandruff, not scalp psoriasis or eczema.

8

The Last Piece of the Puzzle

Since I've been on what is now Psorclear and I've experienced its effectiveness long term, I have been able to find some things to be very true. They have been theorized in many studies. I'm not quite sure if they've ever been substantiated, due to the fact that with the medications that are available that there has never quite been a way to stabilize psoriasis for an extended period of time, in the way and for the length of time that I have been able to stabilize it. It would take that to occur, in order to determine which outside conditions and influences affect psoriasis. Now that I have been able to stabilize and virtually eliminate my psoriasis and know what I do, I definitely do minimize, to the best of my ability, the rare and minor psoriasis flare ups that I do have, to a lesser extent than they ever did years ago. To do more however, would take a lifestyle change that I choose not to pursue right now. As they say, you can't teach an old dog new tricks, unless it wants to learn. The need to do that is now less than it ever was.

I have found that what most drastically aggravates flare ups is alcohol. I do drink alcohol but, not excessively. When those situations do arise and they occasionally do, I will usually get a flare up of my psoriasis, the very next day. As I've said, they are minute in comparison to in the past. The more alcohol I consume, the worse the flare up. If I drink no alcohol at all or, very little as I do now, the flare ups subside. Even the slightest amount of alcohol has an effect on my psoriasis. It's that simple. It appears, at least from my experience, everything that has been said and written about the correlation between alcohol and psoriasis outbreaks is actually very true.

In the past, I also noticed that my psoriasis flare ups will most likely occur when I have a sudden gain in body weight. When that did occur, I didn't increase the amount of zinc or, later on Psorclear that I now take so, I do not know if that would have compensated. I suspect that it might, due to what I mentioned earlier about metabolism and that the amount I took was related to my weight or normal weight. My primary reason for not increasing the dosage, at that time, was that I used it as an incentive to lose weight. It worked for me. I have always been normally heavier in the winter, due to less physical activity. In the last year or so, my physical activity has come almost to a stand-still, primarily due to the pandemic that we're all now dealing with. The good thing is, due to my heart condition, I am on a diuretic that virtually eliminates the possibility of me gaining weight.

As for any special diet, even with the heart condition I have, I am not now, nor have I ever been, on any type of restricted or special diet, nor have I ever put myself on any type of special diet for my psoriasis. I have never been on any type of specialized diet for any of my other medical conditions either. Throughout all my medical issues, at times I have both lost substantial weight and gained substantial weight (over 60 lbs.). Now, because of the medications I take, my weight is fully stabilized and has been for several years now. While going through all my medical issues, neither my psoriasis, nor my zinc intake with Psorclear, was ever once a serious issue. I have stayed clear and never had any flare ups, other than the occasional minor occurrences as mentioned earlier.

Now for the diets...Diets, diets, diets. There are thousands of them. Diets to lose weight, diets to gain muscle mass, lowering cholesterol, for anxiety, diets for one issue or another. Take your pick. Needless to say, there are diets for both psoriasis and eczema. While some are good, some are bad and some virtually do nothing. What I find the most interesting, while reading about diets for psoriasis and eczema, is that a lot of them include foods that are known to be very high in zinc. Hmmm…interesting. Unfortunately, those foods that are high in zinc will not provide enough of the mineral to compensate for any deficiency that you most likely have, as I said earlier in the book.

There are many, many books out there as well as those who say that certain foods may have a therapeutic effect for both psoriasis and eczema. I have never personally found that my diet had anything to do with it since I have been using Psorclear or, the zinc tablets that I first used before Psorclear was formulated. Some of those people may be right but, needless to say, not ever having dealt with a special diet of any kind, I really don't know. It would be up to you to decide what's best for you.

Here are some foods that are high in zinc content but are not enough to help us with our mineral deficiency:

Foods & Nuts:

1. Almonds
2. Beans
3. Beef
4. Cashews
5. Cheese
6. Chicken
7. Chickpeas

Foods & Nuts (Cont.):

8. Crab
9. Lamb
10. Lobster
11. Oysters
12. Pork
13. Pork
14. Pumpkin Seeds
15. Whole Grains
16. Yogurt

Fruits:

1. Apricots
2. Avocados
3. Bananas
4. Blackberries
5. Cantaloupe
6. Dates
7. Dried Figs
8. Kiwi
9. Plantain
10. Pomegranate
11. Prunes
12. Raisins
13. Raspberries
14. Strawberries
15. Tangerine

All I know is that there has never been any type of diet that had any effect, either good or bad, on my psoriasis. I am not a picky eater, by any stretch of the imagination, and I do eat a lot of things people say are not good for you. I like those foods.

Stress always more noticeably took its toll, as I wrote about earlier, although not to the extent that it ever did before I started taking Psorclear. Before, I could never determine whether it was stress or the fact that my current medication had just stopped working. Remember, any flare ups that I have experienced, from time to time, now pale in comparison to the flare ups that occurred before I began taking Psorclear regularly.

As I mentioned in Chapter One, I am a real estate developer and, at the age of 72, I'm trying to figure out why I still am one. This is not a low stress occupation. It is not nearly as stressful as some that I can think of but, never the less, it is very stressful at times. When I am under prolonged stress, which is fairly unusual these days, the flare ups again occur. I guess experience does count for something, even when it comes to dealing with psoriasis. When the stress subsides, so do the flare ups. I am also a very even-tempered person so, the stress levels that I endure are not related to any emotional outbursts. Though I would suspect that would have the same effect.

There are two things about which I cannot tell you about and the effects they have on my psoriasis. That is smoking and drugs (the street variety), for two completely different reasons. I do not use drugs and never have but, I do smoke cigarettes and have since I was about 15, although I am trying to quit, just like everyone else who smokes. I once quit for about two and a half years, back when I had cancer surgery, and I honestly never noticed any difference at that time. That was about fourteen years ago. It is very possible that both could have an adverse effect on psoriasis, since they both take a toll on your metabolism and can have a devastating effect on your body, in general.

I would suspect that, if I did not smoke, it just might help. Although it has never, to my knowledge, been a hindrance. I would also guess that not using drugs would obviously be of help. That however, will always remain a mystery and unknown to me. I also never increased the dosage, back in the day, to see if that would compensate for my smoking.

One thing that I did mention earlier but, only about my scalp, is the effect of sunlight on the psoriasis on the rest of my body, since I began taking what is now Psorclear. The reason I have not is because there are only two words I can say that describe the sun's effect...it helps. It has always helped, in moderation. I'm talking here about natural sunlight, not type of Puva (UVA/UVB treatments with the psoralens). That is a completely different story and, as I mentioned earlier, it only worked for a while and made me sick. The only difference now is that, while it did help a bit before, now I barely even notice because I really don't have any noticeable psoriasis. Most of the spots, which I referred to earlier as minor irritations and blemishes, now just seem to disappear when I spend time in the sun.

In closing, I'm wondering how many of you may remember the old "Sonny and Cher Show", that was on television in the US in the mid-1970s. On that show, they used to have a comedy segment about the "Heartbreak of Psoriasis". You see, "Psoriasis" was this Egyptian princess in the segments and the whole story line was poking fun at the princess. What I don't think they realized, was that there were several million people in the television audience who failed to see the humor. Eventually they must have because, they did remove the segment from the show. To those several million people, the princess "Psoriasis" was not funny. Quite to the contrary, to those people Psoriasis is evil, wicked and has a very nasty sense of humor. Psoriasis wickedly rules the lives of millions of people and is really constantly making all of you miserable and your lives insufferable.

What my friend told me has truly changed my life. Psoriasis is no longer a dirty word and no longer controls me and my life. The wicked princess may not be dead but, at least she is out of my life, for the most part, and no longer controls it. The information that I have shared with you, has changed my life beyond my wildest expectations. There has been a whole lot that I found out in my research over the years. Knowing what I now know and in what I have now passed along to you, your decisions on how to deal with this devastating affliction boils down to just absorbing the related information that is in here and then using common sense. Hopefully that helps you more than what you've been led to believe in the past. I would also sum it up by saying that Psorclear changed my life and gave me hope when nothing else could.

As someone who has really won the war against Psoriasis, I never thought I would be on the winning side of the spectrum. I just had a fading sense of hope that someday, I would find something, just like all of you do. That something for me was what came to be Psorclear, and it could be for you too.

May you get the same benefit from the information in this book as I did. We all deserve it!!

Made in the USA
Middletown, DE
30 December 2021